ELEVATE!

A Journey of Transformation Through Ketamine Therapy

Written By

Jennette B. Boatwright

Table of contents

INTRODUCTION: CLEARING THE WAY TO CHANGE

In the mission for self-awareness and significant change, the human soul continually looks for new roads for height. "Elevate!:A Journey of Transformation Through Ketamine Therapy" is a charming investigation of one such wonderful journey. This book digs profoundly into the universe of Ketamine treatment, a pivotal methodology that has been unobtrusively upsetting the scene of psychological well-being and self-disclosure. Go along with us as we leave on an extraordinary odyssey, directed by the encounters, experiences, and disclosures of people who have navigated the unpredictable territory of their personalities with the guide of Ketamine treatment. Through their accounts, we will uncover the force of this inventive treatment as an impetus for significant self-improvement, recuperation, and the rise of the human soul. "Elevate! " isn't simply a book; it is an encouragement to leave on an expedition of self-revelation, mending, and change, opening the potential inside all of us to transcend life's difficulties and take off higher than ever.

CHAPTER 1: THE FORCE OF KETAMINE TREATMENT: FIGURING OUT ITS BEGINNINGS AND SYSTEMS

In this chapter, we leave on an expedition of revelation into the beginnings and complex systems that support the groundbreaking force of Ketamine treatment. This creative way to deal with emotional well-being and self-improvement has attaches that stretch back to its origin and works through a complicated interchange of neurobiology and brain research.

Ketamine's Introduction to the World and Advancement:

We start by diving into the authentic beginning of Ketamine. Initially blended in the mid-1960s as a sedative specialist, Ketamine was created with the essential point of working with easy medical procedures. Little did its makers have at least some idea that it would develop into a pivotal instrument for psychological wellness change. We follow the medication's change from the working space to the advisor's office, featuring the snapshots of luck and logical investigation that are made ready.

Ketamine's Atomic Dance:

To grasp the force of Ketamine treatment, we should investigate the mind-boggling atomic dance it performs inside the cerebrum. Ketamine's instrument of activity, fundamentally including the glutamate framework, prompts the fast tweak of brain processes. We demystify the neuroscience, offering perusers a reasonable comprehension of how Ketamine can quickly lighten side effects of despondency, tension, and other psychological wellness challenges.

The Hallucinogenic Experience:

Ketamine's belongings stretch out past the physiological domain, offering people a remarkable excursion into changed conditions of cognizance. We dig into the brain research of these encounters, investigating how they can encourage significant bits of knowledge, close-to-home recuperating, and self-awareness. Through the eyes of the individuals who have embraced these journeys, we gain an understanding of the groundbreaking capability of Ketamine-instigated adjusted states.

The Psyche Body Association:

Ketamine's impact isn't bound to the cerebrum alone. Its belongings overflow all through the body, influencing the psyche-body association. We investigate the all-encompassing parts of Ketamine treatment, including its capability to ease actual diseases, improve imagination, and catalyze shifts in discernment that reach out past psychological wellness.

This book fills in as the establishment for our investigation of Ketamine treatment's capability to hoist the human experience. By understanding it is starting points and systems, we are better prepared to see the value in how this creative treatment can clear the way to change and mending, offering desire to those looking for significant change in their lives.

CHAPTER 2: BREAKING THE SHAME: EXPOSING CONFUSIONS ABOUT KETAMINE TREATMENT

Misguided judgments encompassing Ketamine treatment have multiplied, frequently causing some serious qualms about this creative way to deal with psychological well-being treatment. In this chapter, we address and expose probably the most pervasive legends and errors:

Myth 1: Ketamine is Profoundly Habit-forming
The truth:Ketamine treatment is directed in a controlled, clinical setting with exact measurements, making it boundlessly unique about sporting Ketamine use, which is where habit gambles are higher. Various examinations have shown that Ketamine treatment, when regulated capably, doesn't prompt dependence.

Myth 2: Ketamine is Only a Sporting "Party Medication"
The truth: Ketamine has a long history of genuine clinical use as a sedative. Ketamine treatment

includes an alternate setting, with painstakingly oversaw meetings intended to work with mending, self-awareness, and change. It is a long way from being a relaxed party drug.

Myth 3: Ketamine Treatment Is About Mental Trips

The truth : While Ketamine can prompt adjusted conditions of cognizance, the helpful methodology isn't fixated exclusively on dreamlike encounters. These encounters are only one part of the treatment, and the general spotlight is on working with profound contemplation, close-to-home mending, and individual knowledge.

Myth 4: Ketamine Treatment Needs Logical Sponsorship

The truth: Ketamine's viability in dealing with conditions like discouragement and PTSD has been widely contemplated and reported in logical writing. The treatment is supported by thorough examination and clinical preliminaries, making it a deeply grounded treatment choice.

Myth 5: Ketamine Treatment Is a Convenient Solution with No Enduring Advantages

The truth: While Ketamine treatment can make fast impacts, it's anything but a simple "handy solution." Numerous people experience dependable advantages, remembering supported upgrades for mindset, diminished side effects of sadness or nervousness, and improved general prosperity. It tends to be an impetus for significant and enduring change.

Myth 6: Anybody Can Regulate Ketamine Treatment

The truth: Ketamine treatment ought to be regulated via prepared clinical experts or authorized specialists in a clinical or remedial setting. Self-organization or acquiring Ketamine from non-proficient sources is risky and ineffectual.

Myth 7: Ketamine Treatment Is for Everybody

The truth: Ketamine treatment is certainly not a one-size-fits-all arrangement. It may not be reasonable for everybody, and not entirely settled through cautious assessment by medical care suppliers. Individual factors, for example, clinical history and current psychological well-being conditions assume an essential part in deciding office.

Myth 8: Ketamine Treatment is Just About Easing Side Effects

The truth: While side effect help is much of the time an essential objective, Ketamine treatment stretches out past side effects the board. It offers a one-of-a-kind chance for significant self-investigation, close-to-home mending, and self-awareness, making it an important instrument for all-encompassing prosperity.

By dispersing these confusions and giving a more precise comprehension of Ketamine treatment, we mean to cultivate a more open and informed discourse about its capability to change lives and reshape the scene of emotional well-being care

CHAPTER 3: THE SCIENCE BEHIND THE SORCERY: INVESTIGATING THE NEUROBIOLOGY OF KETAMINE'S EFFECT ON PSYCHOLOGICAL WELLNESS

Investigating the neurobiology of Ketamine's effect on psychological well-being is a mind-boggling and continuous interaction that includes a mix of logical exploration techniques.

The following are multiple manners by which specialists examine this significant point:

Animal Studies:

Specialists frequently start by leading examinations on creatures, like rodents, to comprehend what Ketamine means for the mind's neurobiology. These examinations include controlling Ketamine to creatures and afterward analyzing changes in cerebrum science, construction, and conduct. Creature models can give important bits of knowledge into the systems of Ketamine's effect.

Neuroimaging Strategies:

Human examinations oftentimes utilize neuroimaging methods like utilitarian attractive reverberation imaging (fMRI) and positron emanation tomography (PET) filters. These strategies permit scientists to imagine changes in cerebrum action, availability, and construction when Ketamine treatment. Neuroimaging can uncover changes in unambiguous cerebrum locales related to emotional well-being conditions.

Neurochemical Examination:
Analysts break down the degrees of synapses and different neurochemicals in the mind when Ketamine is organized. This incorporates estimating glutamate, serotonin, and dopamine, among others. These examinations give experiences into what Ketamine means for the equilibrium of synapses embroiled in state-of-mind guidelines.

Electrophysiological Studies:
Electrophysiological strategies like electroencephalography (EEG) and magnetoencephalography (MEG) assist analysts with checking cerebrum wave designs and electrical action. Changes in mind motions can be demonstrative of how Ketamine tweaks brain

circuits associated with emotional well-being conditions.

Sub-atomic Science:

Analysts might explore the sub-atomic changes instigated by Ketamine at the cell level. This includes looking at quality articulation, epigenetic adjustments, and the development of proteins associated with synaptic pliancy and neuroprotection.

Clinical Preliminaries:

Clinical preliminaries including human members are vital for grasping Ketamine's consequences for psychological wellness. These preliminaries cautiously screen people with conditions like gloom, nervousness, or post-horrendous pressure issues (PTSD) previously, during, and after Ketamine treatment. Information from these preliminaries gives significant data about the neurobiological changes related to side effect alleviation.

Longitudinal Investigations:

Long-haul studies are fundamental to assessing the supportability of Ketamine's consequences for psychological wellness. These examinations track members over a drawn-out period, looking at whether enhancements continue and whether there are any drawn-out neurobiological changes.

Creature Models of Emotional Well-being Issues:
A few specialists utilize creature models that reenact psychological well-being problems to concentrate on what Ketamine means for the neurobiology of these circumstances. These models assist with uncovering the hidden components of Ketamine's remedial impacts.

Meta-Examinations and Precise Audits:
Scientists likewise total and dissect information from numerous investigations through meta-investigations and orderly surveys. These techniques take into consideration a complete evaluation of the neurobiological impacts of Ketamine across different examinations and populations.

Investigating the neurobiology of Ketamine's effect on psychological wellness is a multidisciplinary exertion that consolidates bits of knowledge from neuroscience, psychiatry, pharmacology, and brain science. This extensive methodology is fundamental for acquiring a more profound comprehension of how Ketamine can be utilized in the treatment of different emotional well-being conditions.

CHAPTER 4: PLANNING FOR THE EXCURSION: EXPLORING THE UNDERLYING STRIDES OF KETAMINE TREATMENT

Exploring the underlying strides of Ketamine Treatment is a painstakingly organized process intended to guarantee both well-being and viability. Here is a thorough aide on how these underlying advances are normally embraced:

Beginning Discussion:

The excursion starts with an underlying counsel with a certified medical services supplier, frequently a therapist or psychological wellness-trained professional. This counsel fills in as a chance for the person to examine their emotional wellness concerns and investigate whether Ketamine treatment is a reasonable treatment choice.

During this conference, the medical services supplier will ask about the singular's clinical history, past psychological well-being therapies, current meds, and any important way of life factors.

Appraisal and Assessment:

A far-reaching psychological wellness appraisal is directed to assess the singular's ongoing emotional well-being status. This appraisal might incorporate normalized polls and meetings to evaluate the seriousness of side effects and generally speaking mental prosperity.

The medical care supplier will focus on the singular's finding and the degree to which their condition has answered past therapies.

Informed Assent:

Before continuing with Ketamine treatment, the medical care supplier will make sense of the therapy exhaustively, including its likely advantages, dangers, and options.

The singular will be offered more than adequate chance to clarify pressing issues and express any worries before giving informed agree to go through Ketamine treatment.

Clinical Screening:

An exhaustive clinical screening is led to survey the person's actual well-being. This screening recognizes any ailments or prescriptions that might contraindicate Ketamine treatment.

Exceptional consideration is given to variables, for example, heart well-being, pulse, and any expected cooperation with existing prescriptions.

Mental Assessment:

A mental assessment is led to additionally survey the person's psychological wellness and decide the fittingness of Ketamine treatment.

The medical care supplier will investigate the singular's therapy objectives and assumptions, assisting with fitting the treatment plan to their particular necessities.

Improvement of a Treatment Plan:

In light of the evaluations and assessments, the medical care supplier, frequently in a joint effort with a psychological wellness group, will foster a customized therapy plan. This plan frames the suggested measurements, recurrence of Ketamine meetings, and treatment objectives.

The treatment plan is made with the singular's novel conditions and targets as a main priority.

Arrangement and Training:

Before the principal Ketamine meeting, the individual gets intensive training on what's in store during therapy. This incorporates data about the likely impacts of Ketamine, both physical and mental.

Methodologies for dealing with any mental inconvenience or difficulties that might emerge during meetings are examined.

Treatment Meetings:

Ketamine treatment regularly includes a progression of meetings directed in a controlled and managed clinical setting. The strategy for the organization (e.g., intravenous implantation, intramuscular infusion, or nasal shower) will rely upon the treatment plan.

During every meeting, the individual gets a painstakingly estimated portion of Ketamine while being firmly checked by prepared medical care experts.

Incorporation and Backing:

Following every Ketamine meeting, people might take part in coordination meetings with a specialist or guide. These meetings give a space to process and incorporate any bits of knowledge, feelings, or encounters that arise during treatment.

Ceaseless help and directing are essential to the remedial cycle.

Checking and Change:

The singular's advancement and reaction to Ketamine treatment are consistently observed. Changes following the treatment plan might be made as important to streamline results.

After Effects, unfavorable responses, or changes in emotional wellness side effects are painstakingly followed and tended to.

Proceeded with Care:

Ketamine treatment is in many cases only one part of an extensive emotional well-being treatment plan. People might go on with different types of treatment, directing, or medicine on the board as suggested by their medical care supplier.

CHAPTER 5: THE KETAMINE EXPERIENCE: UNCOVERING THE EXTRAORDINARY POSSIBLE INSIDE THE HALLUCINOGENIC DOMAIN

Leaving on a journey into the hallucinogenic domain is a significant and groundbreaking experience that can offer profound bits of knowledge, self-awareness, and otherworldly arousing.

To uncover the groundbreaking potential inside this domain, think about the accompanying advances and bits of knowledge:

Set and Setting:

Begin by cautiously picking your set (mentality) and setting (actual climate). A positive and open outlook, liberated from uneasiness or opposition, can work with a more significant encounter.

Make a protected and open setting where you can completely unwind and give up. Guarantee you are in a space liberated from interruptions and possible unsettling influences.

Goals:

Set clear aims for your journey. What do you expect to acquire from this experience? Whether it's mending, self-revelation, innovativeness, or profound knowledge, goals can direct your journey.

Picking the Substance:

Assuming you decide to investigate hallucinogenics, research and pick a substance that lines up with your objectives and solace level. Some notable hallucinogenics incorporate psilocybin (wizardry mushrooms), LSD, and DMT.

Guarantee you are very much informed about the substance's belongings, dose, and expected gambles.

Sitter or Guide:

Consider having a trusted and experienced sitter or guide present during your excursion, particularly on the off chance that you are unpracticed or investigating higher portions.

They can offer close-to-home help, guarantee your security, and assist you with exploring testing minutes.

Care and Contemplation:

Integrate care and contemplation rehearses into your excursion. These strategies can assist you with remaining present, lessen nervousness, and develop your experience.

Zeroing in on your breath and noticing your contemplations and sensations can prompt significant bits of knowledge.

Give up and Giving up:

Embrace giving up on the experience. Relinquish the need to control or direct the excursion. Believe that the hallucinogenic experience will unfurl as it ought to.

Giving up can prompt a more profound association with the psyche and a more extraordinary encounter.

Inward Investigation:

Give close consideration to your viewpoints, feelings, and sensations as they emerge. Investigate the inward scenes of your psyche and heart.

Be available to experience parts of yourself that you might have been staying away from or stifling.

Joining:

After your excursion, carve out an opportunity to reflect and incorporate the bits of knowledge and encounters you acquired. Journaling, workmanship, or conversations with a specialist or guide can support this cycle.

Recognize down-to-earth advances you can take in your day-to-day existence to apply the examples got the hang of during your excursion.

Local area and Backing:

Interface with a strong local area of similar people who have had comparable encounters. Sharing and examining your excursion with others can give approval and knowledge.

Search out assets, books, and associations that advance protected and dependable hallucinogenic use.

Regard and Wariness:

Move toward the hallucinogenic domain with deference and wariness. Comprehend that these encounters can be serious and genuinely testing.

If you have a past filled with psychological wellness issues, counsel a medical care proficient before setting out on a hallucinogenic excursion.

Uncovering the extraordinary potential inside the hallucinogenic domain is a profoundly private and holy jaunt. It requires cautious readiness, expectation setting, and capable use. When drawn closer to veneration and care, this domain can offer significant experiences, mending, and self-improvement. Recollect that security and mindful use are principal, and consistently focus on your prosperity all through the excursion.

CHAPTER 6: RECONCILIATION: SADDLING THE ILLUSTRATIONS AND EXPERIENCES FROM KETAMINE TREATMENT IN REGULAR DAILY EXISTENCE

Ketamine treatment can offer significant experiences and self-improvement. To incorporate the illustrations and bits of knowledge acquired from these groundbreaking encounters into your day-to-day routine, follow these means:

Reflect and Diary:
After every Ketamine treatment meeting, find an opportunity to think about the bits of knowledge, feelings, and considerations that emerged during the experience.
Keep a diary where you can record these reflections. This diary will act as a significant asset for returning to and figuring out your excursion's examples.

Heedful help:
Keep drawing in with a specialist or emotional well-being proficient who has learned about Ketamine treatment and its likely advantages.

Ordinary treatment meetings can assist you with handling your encounters, incorporating bits of knowledge, and working through any difficulties that might emerge.

Solid Way of Life Decisions:
Focus on actual prosperity by keeping a solid eating regimen, ordinary activity, and sufficient rest. Actual well-being can essentially affect mental and profound versatility.
Keep away from substance misuse or unreasonable liquor utilization, as these can impede your capacity to coordinate experiences and keep up with prosperity.

Establish a Strong Climate:
Encircle yourself with a steady and grasping interpersonal organization. Share your encounters and experiences with companions friends and family who can give consolation and sympathy.
Consider joining support gatherings or networks zeroed in on the hallucinogenic mix and emotional wellness.

Put forth Practical Objectives:

Take the bits of knowledge acquired during Ketamine treatment and interpret them into noteworthy objectives in your regular daily existence. These objectives could connect with self-improvement, connections, profession, or imaginative pursuits.

Separate bigger objectives into more modest, feasible moves toward work with progress.

Practice Self-Empathy:

Be thoughtful and patient with yourself as you explore the joining system. Comprehend that development and change require some investment.

Treat mishaps or difficulties as any open doors for learning and development instead of as disappointments.

Innovative Articulation:

Take part in imaginative exercises that permit you to communicate and deal with your feelings and experiences. Workmanship, music, composing, or some other inventive outlet can act as a strong method for reconciliation.

Ordinary Registrations:

Plan ordinary registrations with your psychological well-being proficient to evaluate your advancement, examine any difficulties, and refine your coordination systems.

These registrations can assist with guaranteeing that you are taking advantage of your Ketamine treatment experiences.

Be Available to Change:

Embrace the progressions that normally emerge from your Ketamine treatment encounters. Comprehend that self-improvement might prompt changes in values, needs, and viewpoints.

Adjust and stream with these changes, staying open to additional opportunities.

Keep up with Congruity:

Think about occasional Ketamine upkeep meetings, as suggested by your medical services supplier, to support and develop the bits of knowledge acquired during treatment.

These meetings can assist you with remaining associated with the extraordinary capability of Ketamine treatment.

Bridging the examples and bits of knowledge from Ketamine treatment in regular daily existence is a continuous cycle that requires commitment and care. By incorporating these encounters into your everyday daily practice and looking for help when required, you can keep on developing self-awareness, versatility, and prosperity.

CHAPTER 7: TRACKING DOWN EQUILIBRIUM: OVERSEEING PSYCHOLOGICAL WELLNESS CONDITIONS THROUGH KETAMINE TREATMENT

Arrangement 1: Ketamine Treatment Journaling

One compelling method for overseeing psychological well-being conditions through Ketamine Treatment is to keep a diary. Empower people going through Ketamine Treatment to routinely write down their viewpoints, sentiments, and encounters during and after every meeting. This can assist them with following advancement, recognizing examples, and gaining a more profound comprehension of their emotional wellness.

Guidelines:

Put away a particular time every day to write in your diary.

Record the date and season of your Ketamine Treatment meeting.

Depict how you felt before the meeting (e.g., restless, discouraged, pushed).

Archive your considerations, feelings, and any actual sensations during the treatment meeting.

After the meeting, note any quick changes in your mindset or mental state.

Proceed to diary for a little while or months to notice long-haul impacts.

Arrangement 2: Careful Ketamine Combination

Care methods can supplement Ketamine Treatment, assisting people with dealing with their psychological well-being all the more. Support care rehearses previously, during, and after treatment meetings to upgrade the general insight.

Guidelines:

Before the Ketamine Treatment meeting, practice profound breathing activities to quiet your psyche.

During the meeting, center around your breath or a particular mantra to remain grounded.

After the meeting, require a couple of moments to ponder and consider your encounters.

Use care procedures in your day-to-day routine to oversee pressure and nervousness.

Arrangement 3: Way of life Changes

Overseeing emotional well-being conditions through Ketamine Treatment may likewise include making positive way of life changes. Urge people to embrace sound propensities that can supplement the treatment.

Guidelines:

Begin a workout daily practice: Participate in normal active work, like strolling, running, or yoga, to support your temperament and decrease tension.

Work on your eating routine: Spotlight on a fair eating regimen wealthy in natural products, vegetables, and entire grains while diminishing handled food sources and sugar.

Focus on rest:

Lay out a reliable rest plan and make a loosening up sleep schedule.

Diminish pressure:

Consolidate pressure-decrease strategies like care, contemplation, or profound breathing into your day-to-day daily practice.

Look for social help:

Associate with loved ones, or consider joining support bunches for individuals with comparable emotional wellness challenges.

Arrangement 4: Objective Setting and Progress Following

Setting explicit, feasible objectives and following advancement can be engaging for people going through Ketamine Treatment. Urge them to lay out private objectives connected with their emotional well-being.

Guidelines:

Distinguish at least one psychological well-being objective (e.g., decreasing tension, further developing state of mind, expanding inspiration).

Separate every objective into more modest, sensible advances.

Consistently observe your headway and make adjustments on a case-by-case basis.

Commend your accomplishments, regardless of how little they might appear.

Share your objectives and progress with a specialist or encouraging group of people for added responsibility.

Arrangement 5: Customary Treatment Meetings

Ketamine Treatment can be best when joined with customary talk treatment or directing. Urge people to proceed or begin treatment close by their Ketamine meetings for far-reaching psychological well-being support.

Guidelines:

Find a certified specialist or guide who works in your particular psychological well-being condition.

Plan normal treatment meetings to examine your encounters and feelings.

Team up with your specialist to put forth treatment objectives and keep tabs on your development.

Be transparent during your treatment meetings to amplify their viability.

Recollect that overseeing psychological wellness conditions is a customized excursion, and what works for one individual may not work for another.

CHAPTER 8: PAST ONESELF: KETAMINE TREATMENT'S JOB IN ASSOCIATION, SYMPATHY, AND AGGREGATE RECUPERATING

Ketamine treatment can assume a critical part in encouraging association, empathy, and aggregate mending, principally through its effect on people and the potential for more extensive cultural change. Here is a breakdown of its part there:

1. **Association**:

Upgraded Self-Association: Ketamine treatment, when controlled in a remedial setting, can prompt significant contemplative encounters. It permits people to associate with stifled feelings, recollections, and parts of themselves they might have been keeping away from. This self-association can prompt expanded mindfulness and self-acknowledgement.

Worked on Relational Association:
Through the remedial interaction, people might foster a more profound comprehension of their feelings and ways of behaving, prompting further developed correspondence and association with

others. This can bring about better connections and more noteworthy compassion.

Profound Association:
A few people report encountering a feeling of solidarity or interconnectedness during ketamine encounters, which can cultivate a sensation of association with an option that could be more significant than themselves, whether it's tendency, mankind, or the universe.

2. **Sympathy**:
Self-Sympathy:
Ketamine treatment can help people face and interact with troublesome feelings and self-analysis. This can prompt expanded self-sympathy and a seriously sympathetic mentality towards themselves.

Sympathy Advancement:
Ketamine treatment might improve a singular's ability for compassion by permitting them to investigate their profound profundities. This freshly discovered sympathy can reach out to other people, prompting a more empathetic and figuring out way to deal with relational connections.

Sympathy for Aggregate Mending: As people experience individual recuperating and development through ketamine treatment, they might turn out to be more persuaded to add to the aggregate prosperity of society. Sympathy for others' battles and enduring can drive people to participate in demonstrations of administration, support, or local area building.

3. **Aggregate Recuperating**:

Diminishing Shame:

Ketamine treatment can add to the destigmatization of psychological wellness conditions. At the point when high-profile people transparently talk about their positive encounters with ketamine treatment, it can urge others to look for help unafraid of judgment.

Progressing Psychological Well-being Mindfulness: The examples of overcoming adversity and exploration encompassing ketamine treatment can bring issues to light about the adequacy of elective medicines for psychological wellness conditions. This can prompt more inescapable acknowledgment of imaginative ways to deal with emotional wellness care.

Supporting Foundational Change:
People who go through ketamine treatment and experience individual mending might become advocates for fundamental changes in mental medical care. They might push for further developed admittance to emotional wellness administrations, protection inclusion, and more extensive treatment choices.

CONCLUSION

CHAPTER 9: KETAMINE TREATMENT ENCOUNTERS

Ketamine treatment encounters can differ from one individual to another, yet numerous people report huge positive changes after going through ketamine treatment. A few normal encounters include:

1. Easing of Side Effects:

Ketamine treatment has been demonstrated to be powerful in diminishing side effects of sadness, nervousness, PTSD, and other psychological wellness conditions. Numerous people report feeling a decrease in burdensome considerations, diminished uneasiness levels, and worked on generally speaking temperament.

2. Improved Close-to-Home Mindfulness:

Ketamine treatment can assist people with acquiring a more profound comprehension of their feelings and the fundamental reasons for their psychological wellness battles. Many individuals portray feeling more in contact with their feelings and more equipped for handling and communicating them in better ways.

3. Expanded Knowledge and Clearness:

Ketamine treatment frequently achieves significant experiences and a feeling of lucidity. It can assist people with acquiring another point of view on their lives, connections, and thought processes and conduct. This expanded understanding considers self-improvement and can prompt positive changes in different everyday issues.

4. Otherworldly or Extraordinary Encounters:

A few people report encountering profound or supernatural states during ketamine treatment. These encounters can fluctuate generally, going from sensations of significant association with oneself, others, or the universe, to a feeling of extended cognizance and mindfulness.

5. Profound Delivery:

Ketamine treatment can once in a while set off close-to-home delivery, as people might process and relinquish put away injury or unsettled feelings. This can prompt a feeling of therapy and help.

6. Further developed Connections:

Ketamine treatment can assist people with acquiring their very own superior comprehension needs and limits, which can prompt better and additional satisfying connections. It might likewise empower people to impart all the more successfully and compassionately, encouraging further associations with others.